Anal Fistula Treatment

All you need to know

Dr. Sheila Harrison

Disclaimer

This content serves to provide general information about the disease and aims to empower you to seek prompt medical assistance if necessary to prevent complications. It's essential to stress that this information is not a substitute for consulting a qualified physician. The field of medical science is continually evolving, and due to the dynamic nature of medical knowledge, we recommend seeking expert advice if you encounter any inconsistencies or intend to take action based on the information in this content. Never disregard professional medical guidance or delay treatment based on something you've read online, including this material, or from any other online source. Always remember that the internet cannot cure you; rather, healing comes through the guidance of medical professionals and the providence of God.

Table of contents

Section 1

Introduction

An anal fistula is a condition that affects the anal canal, which is a tube-like structure connecting the rectum to the anus. This medical issue manifests as a small tunnel or channel forming between the skin surrounding the anus and the interior of the anal canal. Typically, anal fistulas arise from infections or abscesses in the anal glands or ducts. The infection often originates in the anal glands, which are tiny structures found within the anus. As the infection progresses, it can lead to the accumulation of pus, which may extend into the adjacent tissues, creating a cavity. Over time, this cavity can evolve into what is known as an anal fistula.

The appearance of an anal fistula is typically characterized by a small opening or orifice in the vicinity of the anus. This condition can be associated with various symptoms, including pain, swelling, and the discharge of bodily fluids. The discharged material may comprise pus, blood, or even fecal matter, and it can emit an unpleasant odor. In certain instances, an anal fistula may be situated deeper within the anal canal, making it less visible from the external surface.

Anal fistulas can be a source of discomfort and concern for individuals experiencing them. If you suspect you have an anal fistula or are dealing with any of the associated symptoms, it is advisable to seek medical attention for proper diagnosis and treatment.

Section 2

Fistula Symptoms

Patients can have different symptoms depending on which parts of the body are connected by the fistula.

Fistula between the small and large intestine

- Diarrhea
- Passage of undigested food

Fistula between the intestine and the bladder

- Urinary tract infection
- Burning with urination
- Cloudy urine or blood in the urine

Fistula between the intestine and the vagina

- Passage of gas or stool through the vagina

Fistula from the intestine to the skin

- Can initially present as a painful bump or boil
- Skin abscess that is open and draining fluid or stool

Section 3

Causes of Anal Fistulas

Most anal fistulas have their origins in anal crypts, which become infected, often leading to the formation of an abscess. When the abscess is incised or spontaneously bursts, it results in the creation of a fistula. An anal fistula can be quite complex, with multiple additional tracts further complicating its anatomical structure.

Other factors contributing to the development of anal fistulas include:

- Opened perianal or ischiorectal abscesses that spontaneously drain through these fistulous tracts.
- Presence of inflammatory bowel disease, particularly Crohn's disease.
- Association with diverticulitis.
- Occurrence due to foreign-body reactions.
- Conditions like
- Actinomycosis
- Chlamydia
- lymphogranuloma venereum (LGV)
- Syphilis

- Tuberculosis.
- Exposure to radiation.
- HIV disease, where approximately 30% of patients develop anorectal abscesses and fistulas.

Section 4

Classifications of Anal Fistulas

Anal fistulas are classified into the following four general types:

Intersphincteric:

Through the dentate line to the anal verge, tracking along the intersphincteric plane, ending in the perianal skin

Transsphincteric:

Through the external sphincter into the ischiorectal fossa, encompassing a portion of the internal and external sphincter, ending in the skin overlying buttocks

Suprasphincteric:

Through the anal crypt and encircling the entire sphincter, ending in the ischiorectal fossa

Extrasphincteric:

Starting high in the anal canal, encompassing the entire sphincter and ending in the skin overlying the buttocks

Section 5

What are the treatment options for anal fistula?

Treatment of anal fistulas depends on

1. The severity of the condition
2. The location of the fistula
3. Evidence of sepsis or a large abscess, or
4. Worrisome findings on physical examination.
5. The underlying cause.

Several treatment options are available, including medications, surgery, and lifestyle changes. You must consult with a healthcare professional, such as a colorectal surgeon, for an accurate diagnosis, classification, and appropriate management of anal fistulas. A specialist can assess the specific characteristics of the fistula and tailor a treatment plan that suits the individual patient's needs.

If an abscess is present, drainage is indicated. Intravenous antibiotics, antipyretics, and analgesics are provided as needed. However, simple rectal abscesses do not typically need antibiotics. [22] If the patient also has sepsis, intravenous fluids or a pressor may be necessary. Depending on the presence of systemic symptoms and the condition of the patient, surgery may be necessary.

For anal fistulas, outpatient follow-up with a surgeon is indicated if consultation did not take place at the time of presentation. Surgical therapy is often indicated for healing of an anal fistula. The surgical approach is dependent on whether the fistula is simple or complex, as well as the risk of complications such as incontinence. A gastroenterologist should be consulted if inflammatory bowel disease is suspected. Asymptomatic anal fistulas from Crohn disease are not managed by surgery. However, if the patient is symptomatic, surgical management should be considered.

Antibiotics should be reserved for those with overlying cellulitis or those with sepsis. Otherwise, symptomatic treatment with analgesics should be considered.

Section 6

Medications for anal fistula treatment

Doctors often prescribe medications as a first-line treatment for anal fistulas. But they alone are generally not sufficient for treating an anal fistula.

Medications can be used in combination with surgical or other interventions to help reduce symptoms and promote healing. Here are some medications that doctors may prescribe as a part of the anal fistula treatment plan:

Antibiotics

Doctors may prescribe antibiotics to treat or prevent infection. If you have an abscess or if the fistula is due to an underlying infection, your doctor may prescribe you antibiotics before surgery to help clear the infection and reduce the risk of complications.

Pain medications

Your doctor may recommend over-the-counter pain relievers, such as ibuprofen or acetaminophen to help manage pain before or after surgery.

Anti-inflammatory drugs
Nonsteroidal anti-inflammatory drugs (NSAIDs), such as ibuprofen or naproxen, may be used to reduce inflammation and swelling.

Immunosuppressants
In some cases, your doctor may prescribe immunosuppressant medications to help manage underlying medical conditions, such as Crohn's disease or ulcerative colitis. This is because these conditions can contribute to the development of anal fistulas. It is important to follow your healthcare provider's recommendations regarding medication use and dosage and to report any side effects or concerns to your provider. Remember, medications alone are unlikely to be effective for treating an anal fistula, and surgery or other interventions may be necessary to promote healing and prevent complications.

Surgery for anal fistula treatment

Surgery is the most effective treatment for anal fistulas. There are several types of surgical options available, depending on the location and severity of the fistula. The goal of surgery is to remove the fistula and repair any damage to the anal canal.

Section 7

Here are some of the most common surgical options for anal fistula treatment:

Fistulotomy

This is the most common type of surgery for treating anal fistulas. It involves cutting open the fistula tract and allowing it to heal from the inside out. The patient may undergo the procedure under local or general anesthesia. They also may need to wear a dressing or pack in the wound for several weeks to help promote healing.

Seton placement

This is used in the treatment of anal fistulas that are deep in the sphincter complex. In this procedure, the surgeon places a small piece of rubber or silk through the fistula tract and leaves it in place for several weeks or months. This helps to keep the tract open and prevent the formation of new abscesses or fistulas. The seton may be tightened gradually over time to help promote healing.

LIFT procedure

The technique known as "ligation of the intersphincteric fistula tract" (LIFT) necessitates a minor cut in the skin close to the fistula and the formation of a piece of tissue to conceal the opening of the fistula. This approach aids in facilitating the healing process and diminishing the likelihood of a reappearance of the condition. Usually, surgeons perform this procedure with the patient under general anesthesia.

Fibrin glue injection

This is a minimally invasive procedure that involves injecting a glue-like substance into the fistula tract to seal it shut. This can be an effective treatment for simple fistulas, in which there is no abscess or infection.

Advancement flap repair

During this surgical technique, the surgeon extracts a section of tissue from either the rectal or anal canal and deploys it to conceal the opening of the fistula. This action serves to facilitate the healing process and diminish the likelihood of a recurrence. Typically, the procedure is carried out with the patient under general anesthesia.

The specific surgical approach chosen is contingent on factors such as the location, complexity, and severity of the fistula. Additionally, the patient's overall health, medical history, and personal preferences play a role in determining the most suitable surgical method. Having an open and candid discussion with your healthcare provider is vital to making a well-informed decision regarding the most appropriate surgery for your individual circumstances.

Medication Summary

Medications are often recommended as the initial approach to treat anal fissures. These medications include topical nitrates, calcium channel blockers, and onabotulinumtoxinA injections. They work by reducing the tone of the anal sphincter, which, in turn, enhances blood flow to the anoderm.

In cases of anal fistulas, antibiotics may be required, particularly when the patient exhibits systemic symptoms. Utilizing postoperative prophylactic antibiotic therapy for a period of 7-10 days, with medications such as ciprofloxacin and metronidazole, is considered a crucial component in preventing the development of anal fistulas after the incision and drainage of perianal abscesses.

Section 8

Fistula Removal

Fistulas require immediate medical attention to prevent serious infections or other problems from developing. Treatment options include medications, surgery, or both.

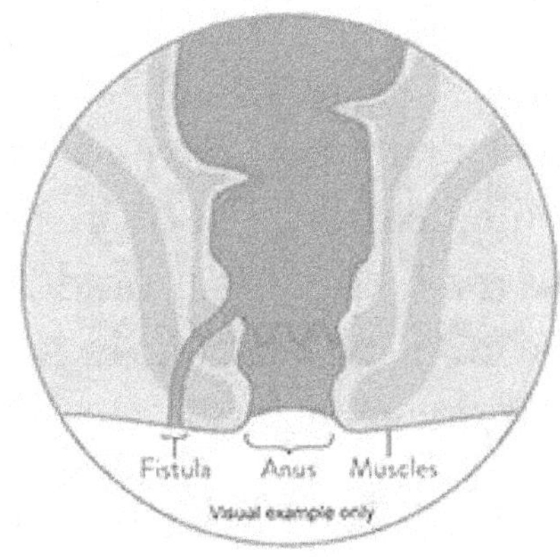

Fistulas form when inflammation causes sores, or ulcers, to form on the inside wall of the intestine or nearby organs. Those ulcers can extend through the entire thickness of the bowel wall, creating a tunnel to drain the pus from the infected area. An abscess, or a collection of pus, can also cause a fistula to form.

The most common types of fistulas in Crohn's disease patients form between two parts of the intestine, between the intestine and another organ, such as the bladder or vagina, or through to the skin surface. Women with Crohn's disease can also develop a fistula between the rectum and vagina, which may be difficult to treat. Surgical treatment depends on individual circumstances.

Fistulas sound scary, but they are treatable. About 35 to 50 percent of adults with Crohn's disease will develop a fistula at some point.

What You Should Know About Fistula Removal

While some fistulas can be treated with antibiotics and other medication, fistula removal surgery may be necessary if the infection doesn't respond to medication or if the fistula is severe enough to require emergency surgery.

There are several surgical options to treat fistulas, including:

- A medical plug to close the fistula and allow it to heal
- A thin surgical cord, called a seton, placed into the fistula to help drain any infection and allow it to heal
- Opening up the fistula with an incision along its length to allow it to heal
- Medical glue to close the fistula

Ileostomy

Your stool will sometimes need to be diverted from the intestine while it's healing from fistula surgery. This is done with an ileostomy, a procedure that brings the small intestine up through the abdominal wall so that waste can leave your body through a surgically created hole called a stoma.

- Feces are collected outside your body in an ostomy pouching system.
- An ileostomy is often used as a temporary solution to allow healing.
- You may require additional surgery to ensure the intestine is closed at the fistula location.

Anal Fistula Removal

An anal fistula is a tunnel that forms between the inside of the anus and the skin surrounding the anus. This is often repaired with a surgical procedure called a fistulotomy.

- The primary goal is to repair the fistula without damaging the anal sphincter muscles, which are necessary for fecal continence, the ability to hold fecal material in your rectum.

- Recurrence rates for anal fistulas are fairly low after surgery.
- Complications are rare and there is typically little impact on fecal continence.

Ask Your Doctor

- What are my options for fistula removal?
- What preparations will I need to make before my fistula removal surgery?
- What are the potential complications from surgery?
- What kind of restrictions will I have after my surgery?
- How long will it take me to recover from fistula removal surgery?
- How will the surgery affect my diet and bowel movements?
- If I require an ileostomy, how do I care for my ostomy pouch and keep it clean?
- What supplies will I need at home?
- Will I need additional surgeries?

Section 9

Lifestyle changes for anal fistula treatment

In addition to medical treatment and surgical intervention, a person can also make certain lifestyle changes to manage the symptoms and promote healing for anal fistulas. Here are some recommended lifestyle changes:

Maintain good hygiene

One of the most important lifestyle changes for anal fistula treatment includes maintaining good hygiene. Keeping the affected area clean and dry is essential for preventing infection and promoting healing. It is recommended to gently clean the area with warm water and mild soap after each bowel movement and to avoid using harsh soaps or perfumes.

Modify your diet

Eating a healthy and well-balanced diet can help promote healing and prevent constipation, which can worsen symptoms and delay healing. Eating foods that are high in fiber, such as fruits, vegetables, and whole grains, and drinking plenty of fluids to stay hydrated is recommended.

Avoid constipation

Constipation can worsen symptoms and delay healing, so it is important to take steps to prevent constipation. This may include eating a high-fiber diet, drinking plenty of fluids, and taking stool softeners or laxatives as directed by your healthcare provider.

Avoid straining during bowel movements

Straining during bowel movements can worsen symptoms and delay healing, so it is important to avoid constipation and take steps to make bowel movements easier. This may include taking stool softeners or laxatives as directed, using a stool or footstool to elevate your feet while on the toilet, and taking your time on the toilet to allow for a complete bowel movement.

Exercise regularly

Regular exercise can help improve overall health and promote healing. It is recommended to engage in regular physical activity, such as walking or swimming, as directed by your healthcare provider.

Quit smoking

Smoking can worsen symptoms and delay healing, so it is important to quit smoking if you are a smoker. Your healthcare provider can provide resources and support to help you stop.

It is important to discuss any lifestyle changes with your healthcare provider before making them, as some changes may not be appropriate for your individual situation. They can help you determine the best approach for managing your symptoms and promoting healing.

In conclusion, anal fistulas are a painful and uncomfortable condition that can be effectively treated with medication, surgery, and lifestyle changes. The treatment options available depend on the severity of the situation, the location of the fistula, and the underlying cause. It is essential to seek medical attention if you experience any symptoms of an anal fistula to prevent complications and promote healing.

Section 10

FAQ on Anal Fistula

Can individuals with diabetes undergo anal fistula treatment?

Yes, diabetic patients can undergo anal fistula treatment. However, they may require additional care and monitoring during the healing process to manage their blood sugar levels effectively, during as well as after the surgery.

Can people with liver or kidney conditions undergo anal fistula treatment?

Yes, people with liver or kidney conditions can undergo anal fistula treatment. However, they may require specialized care and close monitoring to ensure that the procedure is done safely and to manage potential complications.

Is anal fistula treatment safe for individuals with heart conditions?

Anal fistula treatment can generally be performed safely in individuals with heart conditions. However, it is crucial to consult with a cardiologist before undergoing the procedure to evaluate your cardiac health and determine the best course of action.

Is it safe for someone with high cholesterol to undergo anal fistula surgery?

Yes, it is generally safe for individuals with high cholesterol to undergo anal fistula treatment. However, it's crucial to work closely with your doctor to manage your cholesterol levels and follow any necessary dietary and medication guidelines.

What impact does anal fistula treatment have on bone health?

Anal fistula treatment typically does not have a direct impact on bone health. However, it's important for individuals to maintain overall bone health through a balanced diet, regular exercise, and appropriate calcium and vitamin D intake.

www.ingramcontent.com/pod-product-compliance
Lightning Source LLC
Chambersburg PA
CBHW071051260726
48660CB00008B/3171